COURTENAY BETH BOWMAN

Escaping the Narcissist

The Essential Guide to Breaking Free (Safely)

First edition

This book was professionally typeset on Reedsy.
Find out more at reedsy.com

Chuck,

You gently led me out of the fog and into the light. As children we could not understand and as adults we just needed to make sense of things. Thanks for taking the lead and being gentle about it. I'm awake now.

Lizzy Gayle,

I will always be the Thelma to your Louise. Thank you for walking this very long journey with me. It's never boring!

Thelma: "I don't ever remember feeling this awake."

Louise: "You've always been crazy, this is just the first chance you've had to express yourself."

"Bill: [after the tornado passes by them at the drive-in movie theater]

Melissa: I'm saying goodbye.
Bill: No...
Melissa: Sooner or later it would have ended, we both know that. The funny thing is...I'm not that upset. What does that mean?
Bill: I never meant for any of this to happen/Melissa: Oh Billy, I know. It's okay. You go ahead. She needs you.
Bill: What about you?

Melissa: Oh, don't worry about me. I know my way home."

— Dr. Melissa Reeves, Twister

Contents

Preface ii
Acknowledgement iv
1 Understanding Narcissism 1
2 Identifying a Narcissist 5
3 The Impact of Narcissistic Abuse 13
4 Why One Must Leave the Narcissist 19
5 Preparing to Leave 24
6 Executing Your Plan 33
7 Post-Escape Recovery 45
8 Protecting Yourself from Future Narcissists 47
9 Survivor Testimonials 57
10 Legal and Practical Considerations 62
11 Conclusion 67
12 Resources 70
13 Appendix 74
14 References 80
About the Author 82
Also by Courtenay Beth Bowman 83

Preface

The Purpose of **"Escaping the Narcissist"** is to provide an efficient guide for individuals trapped in abusive relationships with narcissists. This book aims to serve as a quick but thorough guide, offering clarity to readers about what narcissistic personality disorder (NPD) is and is not as well as defining narcissistic abuse. Ensuring that possible victims know how to recognize the signs of narcissistic behavior and understand the detrimental impact it can have on their mental, emotional, and physical well-being, individuals can effectively prepare themselves to "break-free" safely from their abuser when and if necessary. By offering practical advice and actionable steps, the first half of this book seeks to empower readers to safely and effectively extricate themselves from the toxic relationship safely and strategically. If you feel trapped and unclear how to break free from your abuser, you will want to focus on the first six chapters of this book. Be smart. You will walk out of this safely, by planning your exit. This is my goal for you and your primary goal right now should only be a safe escape.

Once you have reached safety and caught your breathe, you will be able to begin digesting the second portion of this book. Here you will find support for your recovery and begin your healing process. This section will assist you and any victim in rebuilding your life and protecting yourself from future narcissistic abuse. Through real-life stories, expert insights, and valuable resources, this book aspires to be a beacon of hope and a practical tool for those seeking freedom from the confines of narcissistic manipulation and control. It is designed to immediately offer help for any victim needing to escape from an abusive narcissist. It is also meant to serve as an immediate triage of resources once a survivor has successfully made their escape.

I also want to fully acknowledge, in many cases escaping the narcissist becomes a matter of life and death. Many of us overstay our welcome. We wait too long before we leave. We wait because "of love." We wait until something really bad happens or we wait until our life is threatened and truly on the line or perhaps at least we wait until our "flight response" finally goes off. Perhaps we are waiting for a very clear sign that death will surely come, in vain, or until something inside our gut says, "Oh my god, he is going to kill me." If possible, get out before the life or death moment comes. Not everyone will get to escape.

Eventually, you will get your freedom back. Break-free and heal. There is peace on the other side.

Acknowledgement

To my beautiful adult children who always inspire me and give me a reason to soldier on, Kelsey Elizabeth and Dillon Anthony. You two will always be my most precious gifts and proof of my two-fold recompense.

And to my dearest girlfriend, Pamela Turner, who is more like a sister and who is always there for me, even in the silence you keep me standing, maintain solidarity, and keep perfect vigil over me. I hear you even before the words leave your mouth.

And, of course to my sweet Colonel Houston who built me back up with great ease and without knowing, healed me with his "no nonsense" but sage advice reminding me daily "it's over, move forward."

1

Understanding Narcissism

Narcissistic Personality Disorder (NPD) is a mental condition characterized by a long-term pattern of exaggerated self-importance, a deep need for excessive attention and admiration, history of troubled relationships, and a lack of empathy for others. People with NPD often display arrogance, a sense of superiority, and a lack of consideration for others' feelings. However, many individuals may not have a technical diagnosis for NPD and yet still display narcissistic personality traits such as an inflated sense of self-importance, a deep need for excessive attention and admiration or just a general lack of empathy for others.

Now on the surface, a person displaying traits that may exhibit NPD, may appear to be simply a selfish individual and many people can possess such traits in small doses, but when these characteristics disrupt daily functioning and relationships, or become insidious in nature, or when these characteristics are marked by grandiosity, or a constant need for praise or hypersensitivity to criticism or failure, you could very well be dealing with a narcissist. It is of no consequence whether they have a diagnosis or not.

Key Features of Narcissistic Personality Disorder:

1. **Grandiosity**: An inflated sense of self-importance and superiority over others. This can manifest as boasting, arrogance, and a belief that they deserve special treatment.
2. **Need for Admiration:** A constant need for excessive admiration and validation from others. Narcissists often seek out praise and recognition to reinforce their self-image.
3. **Lack of Empathy:** An inability or unwillingness to recognize or identify with the feelings and needs of others. This leads to insensitivity and exploitation of others for personal gain.
4. **Entitlement:** Belief that they are entitled to special treatment, privileges, and recognition without having to earn them.
5. **Manipulative Behavior:** Using others to achieve personal goals, often through manipulation, deceit, or exploitation.
6. **Fragile Self-Esteem:** Despite their outward **arrogance**, and even haughtiness , narcissists often have a fragile self-esteem and are highly sensitive to criticism or perceived slights.
7. **Envy:** Feelings of envy towards others or belief that others are envious of them.
8. **Interpersonal Issues:** Difficulties in maintaining healthy, mutually satisfying relationships due to their self-centered behavior and lack of empathy.

Diagnostic Criteria:

NPD is diagnosed based on specific criteria outlined in the ***Diagnostic and Statistical Manual of Mental Disorders (DSM-5)***. This Manual is used mainly for therapeutic and insurance purposes. However, remember, there are many narcissists that are never diagnosed as such. Do not let that prevent you from seeking help or safety, or feeling any less mistreated. Remember the diagnostic criteria include that the narcissist has a pervasive pattern of grandiosity, a serious need for admiration, and a lack of empathy, beginning by early adulthood and present in a variety of contexts.

The ***Diagnostic and Statistical Manual of Mental Disorders (DSM-5)*** outlines the criteria for diagnosing NPD. *A person must exhibit at least **five** of the following characteristics:*

1. Grandiose sense of self-importance (e.g., exaggerates achievements and talents, expects to be recognized as superior without commensurate achievements).
2. Preoccupation with fantasies of unlimited success, power, brilliance, beauty, or ideal love.
3. Belief that they are "special" and unique and can only be understood by, or should associate with other special or high-status people or institutions.
4. Requires excessive admiration.
5. Sense of entitlement (i.e., unreasonable expectations of especially favorable treatment or automatic compliance with their expectations).
6. Interpersonally exploitative behavior, taking advantage of others to achieve their own ends.
7. Lack of empathy, unwilling to recognize or identify with the feelings and needs of others.
8. Envious of others or believes that others are envious of them.
9. Arrogant, haughty behaviors or attitudes.

Impact on Relationships:

Individuals with NPD can cause significant emotional and psychological harm to those around them, particularly in close relationships. Their behavior can lead to manipulation, control, and emotional abuse, leaving their partners, family members, and friends feeling devalued and drained.

Understanding NPD is crucial for recognizing the signs of narcissistic behavior and protecting oneself from potential harm. It also highlights the importance of seeking professional help for those affected by or exhibiting symptoms of this disorder.

2

Identifying a Narcissist

Identifying a Narcissist

Recognizing a narcissist early in a relationship can be challenging due to their often charming and charismatic demeanor. However, certain red flags and warning signs can help you identify narcissistic behavior before it becomes too damaging. This chapter will guide you through understanding these signs, recognizing manipulative behaviors, and distinguishing between different types of narcissists.

Red Flags and Warning Signs

1. **Excessive Need for Admiration**
Narcissists constantly seek praise and validation. They may fish for compliments, boast about their achievements, or dominate conversations with stories about their successes.

2. **Grandiose Sense of Self-Importance**
Narcissists often believe they are superior to others and deserve special treatment. They may exaggerate their talents, achievements, or status.

3. **Lack of Empathy**

A key trait of narcissism is an inability or unwillingness to empathize with others. Narcissists are often insensitive to others' feelings and needs and may exploit them for personal gain.

4. **Entitlement**

Narcissists feel entitled to special treatment and often expect others to cater to their needs and desires without reciprocation.

5. **Manipulative Behavior**

Narcissists use manipulation to control and exploit others. They may lie, gaslight, or use guilt to get their way.

6. **Superficial Charm**

Initially, narcissists can be very charming and charismatic. They use their charm to win people over and gain trust.

7. **Inconsistent Behavior**

Narcissists often have a Jekyll-and-Hyde personality. They can be charming and affectionate one moment and cold and cruel the next.

8. **Lack of Accountability**

Narcissists rarely take responsibility for their actions. They often blame others for their problems and refuse to acknowledge their faults.

Early Warning Signs in Relationships

1. **Love Bombing (Typical Narcissist Playbook-Red Flag Warning)**

In the initial stages of a relationship, a narcissist may shower you with excessive attention, affection, and gifts. This "love bombing" is meant to quickly create a sense of dependency and attachment. When a narcissist love bombs a romantic partner, they overwhelm the partner with excessive affection, admiration, and attention in a short period of time. This behavior is often a strategic attempt to quickly establish an intense emotional bond and gain control over the partner. Key characteristics of love bombing include:

1. **Intense Flattery:** Showering the partner with constant compliments and praise, making them feel special and valued.
2. **Frequent Contact**: Bombarding the partner with texts, calls, and messages to maintain constant communication and attention.
3. **Lavish Gifts and Gestures**: Giving expensive gifts or planning extravagant dates and surprises to impress and captivate the partner.
4. **Quick Commitment**: Pushing for rapid progression in the relationship, such as talking about future plans, moving in together, or discussing marriage and children early on.
5. **Idealization**: Putting the partner on a pedestal, idealizing them as perfect and flawless.
6. **Intense Emotional Expressions:** Expressing deep emotions and feelings of love very quickly, often within days or weeks of meeting.
7. **Creating Dependency**: Making the partner feel they are the only source of the narcissist's happiness and fulfillment.

The goal of love bombing is to make the partner feel intensely loved and cherished, creating a sense of dependence on the narcissist for emotional validation. Once the narcissist feels they have secured the partner's affection and trust, they often shift to more manipulative and controlling behaviors, such as gaslighting, emotional blackmail, and devaluation. This cycle can leave the partner confused, emotionally drained, and struggling to regain their sense of self.

2. **Moving Too Fast**

Narcissists often rush the pace of a relationship, pushing for quick commitments or intense emotional bonds early on.

3. **Over-the-Top Flattery**

Narcissists use excessive flattery to make you feel special and valued. However, this can quickly turn into devaluation once they have secured your trust.

4. **Jealousy and Possessiveness**

Early in the relationship, a narcissist may display signs of jealousy and possessiveness, which they may frame as caring or protective behavior.

5. **Testing Boundaries**

Narcissists often test your boundaries early on to see how much control they can exert over you. This may include pushing for things you're uncomfortable with or disregarding your personal *space.*

Manipulative Behaviors and Tactics

1. **Gaslighting (Narcissist "Playbook"-Favorite Tactic)**

Narcissists use gaslighting to make you doubt your perceptions and reality. They may deny things they said or did, twist facts, or make you feel crazy for questioning them.

Gaslighting is a form of psychological manipulation and in the context of a romantic relationship with a narcissist, gaslighting can take several forms:

1. **Denial**: The narcissist denies events or conversations that actually happened, making their partner question their memory.
2. **Trivializing Feelings**: They belittle or dismiss their partner's feelings, suggesting that their emotional responses are irrational or exaggerated.
3. **Blame Shifting**: The narcissist shifts the blame onto their partner for things they themselves did, making the partner feel responsible for the narcissist's actions.
4. **Countering**: They question the partner's recollection of events, insisting that they remember things differently, even when the partner is certain of their memory.
5. **Withholding**: Refusing to engage in conversations or share information, claiming the partner is trying to confuse them or making excuses to avoid discussing important issues.
6. **Discrediting**: They undermine their partner's confidence by suggesting they are forgetful, overly sensitive, or mentally unstable.
7. **Creating Confusion**: The narcissist gives contradictory information or frequently changes their narrative to create confusion and doubt in their partner's mind.
8. **Projection**: Accusing their partner of the very behaviors or traits that they themselves are exhibiting, causing the partner to become defensive and confused.

By employing these tactics, the narcissist seeks to gain control over their partner, eroding their self-confidence and making them increasingly dependent on the narcissist for a sense of reality and self-worth.

2. **Triangulation**

This involves bringing a third person into the relationship to create jealousy, rivalry, or tension. It serves to manipulate you and make you feel insecure.

3. **Projection**

Narcissists often project their own flaws or behaviors onto others. If they are lying or cheating, they might accuse you of doing so to deflect blame and guilt.

4. **Silent Treatment**

When a narcissist feels challenged or slighted, they may use the silent treatment to punish and control you. This withdrawal of communication is meant to make you feel anxious and desperate for their attention.

5. **Guilt-Tripping**

Narcissists use guilt to manipulate you into doing what they want. They may play the victim or accuse you of being selfish to get their way.

6. **Hoovering**

After a breakup or separation, a narcissist might attempt to "hoover" you back into the relationship by making grand promises, apologies, or playing on your emotions.

Different Types of Narcissists

1. **Overt Narcissist**

Overt narcissists are easy to spot due to their blatant arrogance, grandiosity, and need for admiration. They are often charismatic and outgoing, but their self-centeredness and lack of empathy become apparent over time.

2. **Covert Narcissist**

Covert narcissists are more subtle and harder to detect. They may appear shy, humble, or introverted, but they harbor deep-seated feelings of superiority and entitlement. They often use passive-aggressive tactics and play the victim to manipulate others.

3. **Vulnerable Narcissist**

Vulnerable narcissists are hypersensitive to criticism and rejection. They may appear insecure or anxious and are often preoccupied with fears of inadequacy. Despite their vulnerabilities, they still possess a grandiose self-image and a sense of entitlement.

4.Malignant Narcissist: This type combines narcissistic traits with antisocial behaviors, including aggression, paranoia and a lack of remorse. Malignant narcissists are often manipulative and can be dangerous. It should be noted that this type of narcissist is also not found in the Diagnostic Manual under narcissism but the diagnosis is listed under sadism and antisocial behavior. Again, this type of narcissist can be extremely dangerous.

Conclusion

Identifying a narcissist requires careful observation of their behavior and patterns. By recognizing the red flags, early signs, and manipulative tactics, you can protect yourself from falling into a toxic relationships. Understanding the different types of narcissists—overt, covert, and vulnerable and yes even malignant narcissist—will help you discern their behaviors and take appropriate steps to safeguard your well-being. Becoming aware of these traits and behaviors empowers you to make informed decisions about your relationships and take action when needed.

3

The Impact of Narcissistic Abuse

The Impact of Narcissistic Abuse

Narcissistic abuse can have profound and long-lasting effects on victims. This chapter explores the **psychological, emotional, and physical impacts of narcissistic abuse,** including the specific tactic of **gaslighting** and its detrimental effects. We will also examine the social consequences and how relationships deteriorate under the influence of a narcissist.

Psychological Effects

1. **Anxiety and Depression**
   Victims of narcissistic abuse often experience heightened levels of anxiety and depression. The constant criticism, belittlement, and manipulation can lead to feelings of worthlessness and despair. In extreme cases it can lead to thoughts and attempts of suicide.

2. **Post-Traumatic Stress Disorder (PTSD)**
   Repeated exposure to narcissistic abuse can result in PTSD. Symptoms may include flashbacks, nightmares, severe anxiety, and uncontrollable

thoughts about the abusive incidents. Severe abuse can actually change the brain chemistry for the victim of a narcissist. This can actually result in long-term cognitive issues as it relates to basic brain functioning. PTSD has been known to cause disability in victims of severe narcissistic abuse cases where the diagnosis is Complex PTSD after such trauma.

3. **Low Self-Esteem**

Narcissistic abuse can erode a victim's self-esteem. Constant devaluation and criticism can make individuals doubt their worth and capabilities. If you feel bad when you are around the narcissist, this is a good sign that they are chipping away at your self-esteem. This is an excellent litmus test and a good sign that you do not need to be around this individual.

4. **Cognitive Dissonance**

Victims often struggle with cognitive dissonance, where they hold conflicting beliefs due to the narcissist's contradictory behavior. This can lead to confusion, difficulty making decisions, and mental exhaustion. A narcissist counts on keeping you on shaky ground to foster insecurity and ensure dependence. And it is the narcissist who is the one that is constantly clarifying or pretends to clear up any confusion for the victim. This further feeds into the dependency.

Emotional and Mental Health Consequences

1. **Emotional Dysregulation**

Narcissistic abuse can cause victims to experience intense and unpredictable emotions. The abuse disrupts their ability to manage emotions, leading to frequent mood swings and emotional outbursts. This further complicates self-esteem, confusion, and insecurity for the victim.

2. **Guilt and Shame**

Victims often feel overwhelming guilt and shame, believing they are responsible for the abuse or that they deserve it. Unfortunately, victims of narcissists seem to be equal opportunists and narcissists are simply looking for empathic targets that will and are eager to be loved. It is impossible not to be conned by a "love-bombing," manipulative, charming, narcissist. And the narcissist is counting on their victim to feel guilt and shame and enjoys reinforcing these feelings to maintain control.

3. **Hyper-vigilance**

Constantly being on guard to avoid triggering the narcissist's wrath can lead to hyper-vigilance. Victims may become excessively alert to potential threats, leading to chronic stress and anxiety.

4. **Trust Issues**

Experiencing betrayal and manipulation from a narcissist can make it difficult for victims to trust others. This can affect their ability to form healthy, trusting relationships in the future.

Gaslighting and Its Effects

1. **Definition of Gaslighting**

Gaslighting is a manipulative tactic used by narcissists to make victims doubt their perceptions, memories, and sanity. It involves denying, distorting, or fabricating information to create confusion and insecurity. **(Refer to previous Chapter for Gaslighting tactics)**

2. **Impact on Mental Health**

Gaslighting can lead to severe mental health issues, including anxiety, depression, and PTSD. Victims may feel as though they are "going crazy" and ironically become increasingly dependent on the narcissist for validation of reality.

3. **Loss of Confidence**

Constantly doubting their own perceptions and memories can severely undermine a victim's confidence. They may become indecisive and reliant on the narcissist for guidance.

4. **Isolation**

Gaslighting often isolates victims from their support networks. As victims begin to doubt their reality, they may withdraw from friends and family who could offer support and perspective.

Physical and Social Consequences

1. **Impact on Physical Health**

Narcissistic abuse can take a toll on physical health. Chronic stress and anxiety can lead to a range of health issues, including:

- Headaches and migraines
- Gastrointestinal problems
- High blood pressure
- Insomnia
- Weakened immune system

2. **Social Isolation**

Narcissists often isolate their victims from friends, family, and social networks. This isolation increases the victim's dependence on the narcissist and reduces the likelihood of receiving outside support.

3. **Deterioration of Relationships**

Narcissistic abuse can cause significant strain on relationships with others. Victims may become distrustful, withdrawn, or overly dependent, leading to conflicts and breakdowns in communication with loved ones.

4. **Job and Financial Consequences**

The emotional turmoil and mental health issues caused by narcissistic abuse can affect a victim's ability to perform at work, leading to job loss or financial instability. Narcissists may also directly sabotage a victim's career or financial standing.

Isolation and Relationship Deterioration

1. **Emotional Withdrawal**

Victims may withdraw emotionally as a coping mechanism, creating distance in their relationships with friends and family. This withdrawal can lead to feelings of loneliness and abandonment.

2. **Loss of Social Support**

As victims become more isolated, they lose valuable social support networks. This lack of support makes it more difficult to escape the abusive relationship and recover from its effects.

3. **Strained Family Relationships**

Narcissistic abuse often strains relationships with family members. Victims may become estranged from their families due to the narcissist's influence or their own feelings of shame and guilt.

4. **Dependency on the Narcissist**

Isolation increases a victim's dependency on the narcissist, making it harder to leave the relationship. The narcissist may exploit this dependency to further manipulate and control the victim.

Conclusion

The impact of narcissistic abuse is far-reaching and can affect every aspect of a victim's life. From psychological and emotional health to physical well-being and social relationships, the consequences are profound and enduring. Understanding these effects is the first step toward recognizing the need for change and seeking help. By acknowledging the damage caused by narcissistic abuse, victims can begin the journey toward healing and reclaiming their lives.

4

Why One Must Leave the Narcissist

Recognizing and escaping narcissistic relationships is crucial for several reasons:

1. Protecting Mental Health

Narcissistic relationships can be extremely damaging to one's mental health. Narcissists often engage in manipulation, gaslighting, and emotional abuse, leading to anxiety, depression, and diminished self-esteem. Recognizing these relationships early can help prevent long-term psychological harm. The narcissist's behavior is progressive and can only be expected to escalate and become more damaging.

2. **Preserving Emotional Well-being**

Constantly dealing with a narcissist's need for admiration and lack of empathy can be emotionally exhausting. Individuals in such relationships often experience feelings of worthlessness and helplessness. Escaping these toxic dynamics is essential for reclaiming emotional stability and well-being. Escape is the only way to learn interdependence again and exercise self-care. The narcissist loses no sleep knowing you are exhausting yourself by constantly trying to address their personal needs.

3. **Preventing Physical Harm**

In some cases, narcissistic behavior can escalate to physical abuse. Recognizing the signs of a narcissistic relationship can be the first step in protecting oneself from potential physical danger and ensuring personal safety. In many cases the narcissist may also have other addictive behaviors that may escalate issues and exacerbate the narcissistic behavior further such as drug, alcohol, gambling or pornography issues.

4. **Reclaiming Personal Autonomy**

Narcissists often exert control over their partners' lives, making it difficult for them to make independent decisions or pursue their own goals. Escaping these relationships allows individuals to regain their autonomy and pursue their own interests and aspirations.

5. **Improving Quality of Life**

Living with a narcissist can lead to constant stress and tension, affecting overall quality of life. By escaping the relationship, individuals can create a more peaceful and fulfilling environment for themselves, leading to better overall health and happiness.

6. **Promoting Healthy Relationships**

Recognizing and escaping a narcissistic relationship is a critical step towards healing and learning to build healthier relationships in the future. It involves understanding what a healthy relationship looks like and setting appropriate boundaries to protect oneself.

7. **Empowering Personal Growth**

Breaking free from a narcissistic relationship is an empowering act that can foster personal growth and resilience. It helps individuals rediscover their self-worth, build confidence, and develop stronger, healthier coping mechanisms.

8. **Providing a Safe Environment for Others**

For those with children or dependents, escaping a narcissistic relationship is vital to creating a safe and nurturing environment. It prevents the perpetuation of abusive behaviors and ensures that children are not exposed to harmful dynamics.

9. **Accessing Support and Resources**

Recognizing the signs of narcissistic abuse can prompt individuals to seek the necessary support and resources, such as therapy and support groups, which are essential for recovery and rebuilding their lives. Overall, recognizing and escaping narcissistic relationships is essential for safeguarding one's mental, emotional, and physical health. It enables individuals to break free from toxic patterns, regain control of their lives, and move towards healthier, more fulfilling relationships.

In many cases escaping the narcissist becomes a matter of life and death. Many of us overstay our welcome. We wait too long before we leave. We wait until something really bad happens or our life is truly on the line or we wait until our "flight response" finally goes off. Perhaps we wait until something inside our gut says, "Oh my god, he is going to kill me." If possible, get out before that moment.

But, some situations can be so volatile that your only goal will be to escape, to get to safety, and to get away from the narcissist. And, eventually, you will get your freedom back.

(Abusive Tactics) Common Behaviors and Patterns of a Narcissist

1. **Manipulation and Control**: Narcissists often use manipulative tactics, such as gaslighting, to control and dominate their relationships. They distort reality to make others doubt their perceptions and believe the narcissist's version of events.
2. **Lack of Accountability:** Narcissists rarely take responsibility for their actions. They often blame others for their mistakes or shortcomings and refuse to acknowledge their faults.
3. **Excessive Need for Praise:** They constantly seek validation and admiration from others. When they do not receive the attention they crave, they may become upset or angry.
4. **Superficial Charm:** Narcissists can be charming and charismatic, especially in the early stages of a relationship. They use their charm to win people over and gain their trust.
5. **Boundary Violations:** They often disregard personal boundaries and may intrude on others' privacy, possessions, or time without regard for their feelings or consent.
6. **Jealousy and Envy:** Narcissists are often envious of others' success or happiness and may attempt to undermine or belittle those they perceive as a threat.
7. **Isolation Tactics:** They may isolate their victims from friends and family to maintain control and dependence.
8. **Volatile Emotions:** Narcissists can be prone to emotional outbursts, especially when their sense of superiority is challenged. This can include rage, sulking, or giving the silent treatment.

Conclusion

Understanding the characteristics and behaviors associated with narcissism is the first step in recognizing and addressing these toxic dynamics. By learning about the different types of narcissism and the criteria for NPD, individuals can better identify narcissistic traits in their relationships and take appropriate steps to protect themselves. Recognizing these patterns is crucial for safeguarding one's mental and emotional well-being and ultimately escaping the damaging effects of a narcissistic relationship. There is no known cure for narcissism. There are many reasons it is easier and safer to leave and be safe than to confront a narcissist or to expect a narcissist to change.

5

Preparing to Leave

Preparing to Leave the Narcissist

Leaving a narcissistic relationship is a significant and often challenging step. This chapter will guide you through assessing your current situation, evaluating risks and safety concerns, creating a comprehensive safety plan, and understanding legal considerations and resources to ensure both physical and emotional safety.

A. Assessing the Situation

(see Appendix for Self-Assessment of Relationship Health Questionnaire and "Are you Being Abused"? Checklist)

1. **Recognizing the Need to Leave**
Understanding that you are in a toxic and abusive relationship is the first step. Reflect on the impact that the relationship has had on your mental, emotional, and physical health. Acknowledge that leaving is necessary for your well-being and safety.

2. **Understanding the Current Situation**

Take stock of your current circumstances. Consider the following questions:

- How does the narcissist react to conflict or perceived threats?
- Are there patterns of behavior that escalate the risk of violence or manipulation?
- What resources and support systems do you currently have?

3. **Evaluating Emotional Readiness**

Leaving a narcissist is emotionally taxing. Assess your emotional readiness by considering your support network, coping mechanisms, and mental health. Seek therapy or counseling to help bolster your emotional resilience, if there is time and it is safe to do so.

B. Evaluating Risks and Safety Concerns

*Trying to leave a narcissist can be a very dangerous time. Because the narcissist is so unpredictable and rejection is a natural trigger for the narcissist it can be especially volatile. This is why it is critical to have everything well planned out. If the narcissist has additional drug or alcohol issues, this also needs to be an additional consideration when planning your exit. **(See Appendix for Evaluating Risks and Safety Concerns Checklist)**

1. **Identifying Potential Risks**

Narcissists can react unpredictably to rejection or loss of control. Identify/consider potential risks, (and attempt to circumvent any negative outcome if possible by planning for contingencies) including:

- Physical violence or aggression

- Stalking or harassment
- Financial retaliation
- Legal manipulation (e.g., custody battles, false accusations)

2. **Understanding Escalation Patterns**

Recognize behaviors that signal escalation, such as increased anger, threats, or erratic behavior. Understanding these patterns can help you anticipate and mitigate risks.

3. **Considering Dependents**

If you have children or other dependents, evaluate their safety and well-being. Consider how the narcissist's behavior affects them and incorporate their needs into your safety plan.

C. Creating a Safety Plan

(Refer to Appendix for How to Create a Safety Plan)

1. **Establishing a Support Network**

Identify trusted friends, family members, or support groups who can provide emotional and practical support. Inform them of your situation and plan.

2. **Securing Important Documents**

Gather and secure essential documents, such as identification, financial records, legal documents, and any evidence of abuse. Keep copies in a safe place outside the home.

3. **Financial Preparation**

Prepare financially by:

- Opening a separate bank account

- Saving money discreetly
- Keeping track of shared financial assets and debts

4. **Planning for Immediate Safety**

Create a detailed plan for leaving, including:

- Safe places to go (e.g., a friend's house, a shelter)
- Transportation arrangements
- An emergency bag (**see Appendix for Bug-out-bag checklist**) with essentials (clothes, medications, important documents)

D. Steps to Ensure Physical and Emotional Safety

1. **Secure Communication**

Use secure methods of communication to avoid the narcissist's surveillance. Consider using a new phone, email, and social media accounts.

2. **Change Routines**

Alter your daily routines to make it harder for the narcissist to predict your movements. This includes changing routes to work, varying shopping times, and altering other regular activities.

3. **Legal Protection**

Consider obtaining a restraining order or protection order if there is a risk of violence or harassment. Consult with a legal professional to understand your options and the process.

4. **Seek Professional Help**

Engage with professionals such as therapists, counselors, and legal advisors to support your mental health and navigate the legal complexities of leaving.

E. Legal Considerations and Resources

1. **Understanding Your Rights**
   Educate yourself about your legal rights regarding property, finances, and custody. This knowledge empowers you to make informed decisions and protect yourself legally.

2. **Custody and Child Support**
   If you have children, understand the laws surrounding custody and child support. Document any abusive behavior that could impact custody decisions.

3. **Legal Resources**
   Utilize legal resources such as:

   - Domestic violence hotlines and shelters
   - Legal aid organizations
   - Family law attorneys who specialize in domestic abuse cases

4. **Documenting Abuse**
   Maintain detailed records of any abusive incidents, including dates, descriptions, and any evidence (e.g., photos, messages). This documentation can be crucial in legal proceedings.

5. **Restraining Orders**
   Learn about the process for obtaining restraining or protection orders. These legal instruments can provide immediate protection and establish boundaries.

F. Signs Your Partner Might Be Tracking You

***Being tracked is something you may not have considered, but is important to be mindful of in keeping you safe. Determining if your partner is tracking you can be challenging, especially if they are using discreet or covert methods. Here are some signs and steps you can take to find out if you are being monitored:**

1. **Unexplained Knowledge:** Your partner knows your whereabouts, conversations, or activities that you haven't shared with them.
2. **Changes in Behavior:** They suddenly become very controlling or possessive without any clear reason.
3. **Frequent Accusations:** They frequently accuse you of lying or cheating, often citing "proof" or details that seem very precise.
4. **Tech Savviness**: Your partner is very knowledgeable about technology and has access to your devices.
5. **Unusual Device Behavior:** Your phone, computer, or other devices start acting strangely—such as unusual battery drain, increased data usage, or unexpected reboots.
6. **Unexpected Messages or Alerts**: You receive unusual messages, alerts, or notifications that could indicate spyware or tracking apps.

G. Steps to Determine If You're Being Tracked

1.Check Your Devices for Tracking Apps:

- Android: Go to Settings > Apps > All Apps and look for any unfamiliar or suspicious apps.
- iPhone: Go to Settings > General > iPhone Storage and review the list of installed apps. Also, check Settings > Privacy > Location Services to see which apps are using your location.

- Browser History: Check your web browser's history for any visits to websites associated with tracking software.

2.Look for Spyware and Monitoring Software:

- Use reputable antivirus and anti-spyware software to scan your devices for malicious applications.
- Reset your device to factory settings if you suspect it's compromised, but ensure you back up important data first.

3.Examine Physical Tracking Devices:

- Check your car for GPS tracking devices. Look under the dashboard, in the glove compartment, and around the wheels.
- Inspect your personal belongings, such as bags and clothing, for small tracking devices.

4.Review Your Phone Settings:

- Location Services: Ensure location services are turned off or restricted for apps that don't need it. Go to your phone's settings and manage location permissions.
- Sharing Location: Check if you are unknowingly sharing your location through apps like Find My iPhone, Google Maps, or social media platforms.
- Bluetooth and Wi-Fi: Turn off Bluetooth and Wi-Fi when not in use to prevent unauthorized connections.

5.Monitor Your Network Traffic:

- Use network monitoring tools to see if there's unusual data traffic on your devices. High data usage could indicate that information is being sent to a third party.

6.Secure Your Accounts:

- Change your passwords regularly and use strong, unique passwords for each account.
- Enable two-factor authentication (2FA) on your accounts to add an extra layer of security.

7.Get Professional Help:

- Consult with a tech-savvy friend, a professional IT expert, or a cybersecurity specialist if you suspect you are being tracked but can't identify how.

H. Protecting Yourself

- **Use a Safe Device:** If possible, use a device that your partner doesn't have access to for sensitive communications and searches.
- **Seek Support**: Reach out to local domestic violence organizations or hotlines for help. They can provide resources and advice specific to your situation.
- **Legal Options:** Consult with a lawyer about your legal rights and options for protection, such as obtaining a restraining order.

Taking these steps can help you determine if you are being tracked and take measures to protect your privacy and safety.

Final Thoughts

Preparing to leave a narcissist requires careful planning and consideration of various factors to ensure your safety and well-being. By assessing your situation, evaluating risks, creating a detailed safety plan, and understanding legal considerations, you can take proactive steps to protect yourself and your loved ones. Remember that seeking support from trusted individuals and professionals is essential throughout this process. Leaving a narcissistic relationship is challenging, but with preparation and support, you can achieve safety and freedom, paving the way for healing and a healthier future.

6

Executing Your Plan

Executing Your Plan

Leaving a narcissistic relationship requires careful execution to ensure your safety and well-being. This chapter provides practical steps for leaving, financial preparation, finding a safe place to stay, communicating your departure, and handling reactions and potential backlash. Remember you are trying to avoid having events escalate to the point where you must flee, leaving everything behind. This may be your only time for prudent and logical planning. It is best to do this when things have not escalated to a volatile situation. The narcissist is manipulative and their sense of entitlement, arrogance, and lack of empathy will make it extremely difficult to execute even an iron-clad plan if you are not well-prepared.

Practical Steps to Consider Before You Leave

1. **Timing and Logistics**

Choose a time to leave when the narcissist is not around or distracted. Ensure you have a clear plan for where you will go and how you will get there.

2. **Emergency Bag (refer to Appendix for bug-out-bag checklist)**

Prepare an emergency bag with essentials, including clothes, medications, important documents, keys, and some cash. Keep it in a place where you can easily access it when needed. Sometimes this may be difficult. It means that you may have to insist on an extra supply of medication from your doctor, or to ensure that you stash cash without "borrowing" from this stash. It also means it may be best to use travel size items so the narcissist will not notice that certain items are out of the regular rotation of daily life, such as favorite clothing items, your regular toothbrush and the favorite travel bag.

3. **Support Network**

Inform your trusted support network about your plan. Ensure they know how to contact you and can provide immediate assistance if necessary. I cannot stress the importance of keeping your circle small and ensuring that this group of individuals is able to believe and support you. Many shared friends will turn on you in the end, having successfully been manipulated by the narcissist. This also means that during your exit, if you have reached out and trusted the wrong friend, your life may be in even more danger. Not everyone will understand your family dynamic and what you are escaping. Choose wisely and ensure that they will keep your confidence. As you begin thinking about leaving, it is always a good time to condense and scale down your trusted circle of friends.

4. **Transportation**

Arrange reliable transportation to your safe location. This could be a friend or family member, a taxi, or public transportation. Ensure you have a backup plan or contingency plan and always assume that your primary option will be foiled in some way. If you plan for a contingency then under extreme stress, you will be able to flip into your next alternate plan with great ease and without much thinking. This is the goal of being prepared.

5. **Notify Authorities (Community Advocate)**

If you fear for your safety, consider notifying local authorities about your plan. They can provide immediate assistance or be on alert in case of an emergency. Also, most domestic violence shelters have non-residential services to include legal services for both female and male clients at no cost. It is possible to simply "go on record" with your safety plan at most shelters and ensure that you have a good plan in place. It is often an excellent idea to have a community advocate that has a record of you seeking consult during this exit period.

Of course, a shelter is also a good contingency plan if you fear for your safety or it becomes necessary to obtain a safe alternative location were the narcissist to find you. Remember your exit will be one of the most precarious times of your relationship with the narcissist and things may become volatile even if the narcissist has never shown signs of violence in the past. You have rejected them now and it is difficult to predict how the narcissist will react. But remember, a local shelter can assist you with all these resources as a non-residential client.

Financial Preparation and Independence

1. **Separate Finances**

Open a separate bank account in your name if you haven't already. Ensure that any direct deposits or financial resources are directed to this account. Understanding that this might be very difficult, especially if you are married to the narcissist, it may mean that you plan your exit close to a payday when the bank account is low. You may then have to ensure that you cancel your direct deposit, intercept your check and deposit your money in a new bank account that only you have access to from this point.

2. **Save Money Discreetly**

Save money discretely over time. This could involve setting aside small amounts from household expenses or finding additional income sources, like a hobby business, having garage sales, or selling items you are no longer using, or getting and saving small amounts of cash you get back when purchasing groceries at the store.

3. **Understand Your Financial Situation**

Make a detailed list of shared and individual assets and debts. This will be important for future legal and financial decisions. Certainly if you are married, this is one of the more important areas of documentation. Try to take photos of recent statements of all your credit cards bills and statements, so that you have account numbers, ideas of debts, assets, and even the narcissist's personal data for identification purposes, to include SS# and VIN# to the vehicle they might own. Copies of recent tax records and checking and savings account numbers are all important to gather as well.

4. **Seek Financial Advice**

Consult with a financial advisor or legal professional to understand your financial rights and options. They can help you prepare for financial independence. While this is a perfect idea ahead of time, it may not be practical until you have made your break from the narcissist. Alone and on your own, your financial picture will look much different. Sometimes things must "shake out" before a clear financial picture can manifest. You do have rights and if you are married or own a home, you certainly have rights to those assets and both legal and financial advice is prudent in this regard, which is why it is necessary for you to know and have documentation as to what you both possess before leaving.

Finding a Safe Place to Stay

1. **Friends and Family**

Reach out to trusted friends or family members who can offer you a place to stay. Ensure they understand the seriousness of the situation and can provide a safe and supportive environment. Consider you friends' and family's safety as well. If you think that your mother's house is the first place the narcissist will come looking for you, it is probably not safe for you or your mother that you stay with her. Bear this in mind. While it is nice to be close to trusted friends and family, if it will caused additional drama or hardship, be careful to weigh the possible consequences.

2. **Shelters and Safe Houses**

Research local shelters or safe houses for victims of domestic abuse. These places offer not only safety but also resources and support services. As mentioned previously when discussing "Notifying Authorities" and seeking the help of Community Advocates, shelters are viable and important resources and a good alternative.

3. **Long-Term Housing**

Consider your long-term housing options. This could involve looking for rental properties, applying for housing assistance programs, or staying with supportive friends or family until you find permanent accommodation. It is often helpful to seek a period of transition housing after leaving the narcissist. This time is a period of healing, acclimation and will feel like you have just been through a terribly traumatic event. On the other hand, you may also feel completely numb to the entire situation and not prepared to make long term decisions about anything. You may be doing well to take things day by day as long-term planning may feel entirely too overwhelming at this point. Your goal is simply a roof over your head and possibly your children's if applicable and to maintain care for yourself.

Communicating Your Departure

In many cases, it's not necessary—and often not advisable—to communicate your intention to leave to a narcissist. Narcissists can react unpredictably, and informing them in advance can lead to manipulative, controlling, or even dangerous behaviors aimed at preventing your departure.

Instead, focus on preparing your exit plan quietly and ensuring your safety. Seek support from trusted friends, family, or professionals, and have everything in place before making your move. However, if you feel you must communicate your exit here are some of your options:

1. **Written Communication**
   If direct communication is too dangerous, consider writing a letter or email explaining your departure. Be clear, firm, and concise, and avoid engaging in further dialogue. This will basically allow you to tell the narcissist how it is going to be without discussion or the chance to be manipulated into staying.

2. **In-Person Communication**
   If you choose to communicate in person, although very risky, ensure

it is in a public place or have a trusted person present. Be prepared for manipulation or emotional outbursts and stick to your decision. Even if you are in public, do not expect that to save you, especially if you have a trusted person with you. Remember that while you may feel safer with a friend, the narcissist will do almost anything to maintain that feeling of superiority and need for admiration in public. He/she will not take kindly to being shown-up in front of someone else.

3. **Third-Party Mediation**

In some cases, using a mediator such as a therapist or lawyer can help communicate your decision safely and effectively. This adds a layer of protection and objectivity to the situation. This is an excellent choice for those who have the following situations and must consider them:

1. **Shared Responsibilities:** If there are shared responsibilities, such as children, pets, or finances, discussing the departure might be necessary to arrange logistics and ensure continuity of care.
2. **Legal Requirements:** In some cases, legal considerations might necessitate informing the narcissist, such as in situations involving divorce proceedings or custody arrangements.
3. **Safety and Support:** If the person feels safe enough and has a strong support network, they might opt to inform the narcissist to avoid sudden and potentially escalated reactions. This can be risky and difficult to predict. Exercise caution.
4. **Mutual Agreements**: In some relationships, despite the narcissism, there may be a history of mutual agreements where open communication is expected or legally required.

Strategies for Breaking the News

1. **Be Direct and Firm**

Clearly state your decision to leave. Avoid giving false hope or engaging in long explanations. Be direct and firm about your reasons and your plans. You can say something like this in person or even write something similar:

> *"I need to let you know that I am moving out of the house today. I feel emotionally distressed and unsafe here, and this decision is for my own mental health and well-being. Do not contact or follow me or try to find me. You may email me or contact me through my attorney only. If you try to contact me directly, I will be forced to get a restraining order."*

This is clear. It gives you the last word and it also says, you are distressed, feel unsafe and gives the warning that you have an attorney and will take more advanced measures if the narcissist bothers you further by legally obtaining an restraining order.

2. **Prepare for Emotional Manipulation**

Expect the narcissist to use emotional manipulation, such as guilt-tripping, begging, or making promises of change. In fact the narcissist will probably pull out all the stops if they are really desperate and use every trick in their guilt-tripping tool-belt to make you feel responsible for their unhappiness and unmet needs. They will remind you of their past sacrifices, play the martyr, remind you of your shortcomings, flaws and failures, and even exaggerate feelings of hurt and disappointment that you have put them through. This will typically be over ridiculous minor stuff. Do NOT TAKE THE BAIT. The narcissist will use phrases like "If you really really loved me, you would..." just to pressure you. They will be hurtful and compare you unfavorably to others, and they will blame their emotional states on you, telling you that you are causing them to be so angry with you. They will use your personal, most intimate secrets and stories as ammunition now to hurt you. So, be prepared. And, they will accuse you of neglecting them, the relationship, the marriage, the kids, not doing enough to keep them happy and satisfied. It is all manipulation. Stay firm in your decision and remind yourself of the reasons you are leaving.

3. Limit Communication

After breaking the news, limit further communication. Block phone numbers and social media accounts if necessary to avoid harassment and manipulation. If you have no ties, such as a legal commitment or household, or children, employ the **NO CONTACT RULE.** If you are unable to do this then by all means, keep it to a minimum and speak through an attorney if possible.

NO CONTACT RULE - involves completely cutting off all forms of communication and interaction with the narcissist. Here's a breakdown of what it typically entails:

1. **Cease All Communication**: This means no phone calls, text messages, emails, social media interactions, or any other form of contact.
2. **Avoid Physical Contact**: Do not meet in person or go to places where you might encounter the narcissist.
3. **Set Clear Boundaries:** Inform the narcissist that you do not want any contact. If necessary, communicate this boundary through a third party, such as a lawyer.
4. **Block Access:** Block their phone number, email, and social media accounts. Adjust your privacy settings to prevent them from accessing your information.
5. **Handle Shared Responsibilities Separately**: If you have shared

responsibilities, such as children, find ways to manage these without direct contact. Use a third party or legal arrangements to handle necessary interactions.

6. **Seek Legal Protection if Needed:** If the narcissist continues to contact or harass you, consider seeking a restraining order or other legal protections.

*The goal of the no contact rule is to protect your emotional and mental health, allowing you to heal and regain control of your life without the narcissist's influence. It is absolutely designed to protect you and should be employed at all costs. It is the best and quickest way to heal.

Handling Reactions and Potential Backlash

1. Expect a Range of Reactions

Narcissists may react with anger, sadness, threats, or attempts to win you back. Prepare for a range of reactions and plan how you will respond to each. Ideally, you will employ NO CONTACT or have only minimal contact so you will not need to worry about this issue. However, this is why it is important to be well versed in the manipulation tactics of the narcissist. This way you will know to what degree you are being controlled and manipulated. You can expect it and you can recognize it, if you are well versed in the narcissist's tactics.

2. **Safety Measures**

Increase your safety measures after breaking the news. This might include changing locks, installing security systems, or staying with a trusted person for added security. Based on the state you live in, please ensure that you are well versed in the law and what you are able to do legally, in order to protect yourself. And, know your legal rights in the area of self-defense. Local law enforcement should be able to assist you with this information or a domestic violence shelter may also be able to point you in the right direction.

3. **Legal Protection**

Consider obtaining a restraining order if there is a risk of violence or harassment. Give careful consideration if the narcissist uses drugs or alcohol or possesses firearms as well. Only you know the mental state, background, previous or current diagnosis and training/ work history of the narcissist. This is all information that may be important. For example, if a narcissist once worked Special Ops in the military but is now retired and is currently diagnosed with PTSD and owns an arsenal of weapons, this may be important to share. But always, consult with a legal professional to understand the process and requirements. There are times when we miss the obvious because we are right in the thick of things and cannot see. You may also consult a Domestic Violence Shelter or legal aid in your area for more information.

4. **Document Everything**

Keep detailed records of all interactions and incidents after your departure. This documentation can be crucial for legal proceedings and protecting yourself from false accusations. It would probably be best to keep a running tally of interaction in every form with the narcissist to include date, time, mode of contact, tenor (mood), nature of interaction or request in an electronic log that is saved in the cloud so that if something happens to your phone or computer, the record can still be accessed from anywhere.

Conclusion

Executing your plan to leave a narcissist requires careful planning, financial preparation, and securing a safe place to stay. Communicating your departure clearly and handling reactions with firmness and preparedness are key to ensuring your safety and well-being. By following these practical steps, you can take control of your situation, protect yourself from potential backlash, and begin the journey towards healing and independence. Remember, seeking support from trusted individuals and professionals is essential throughout this process. If you have health insurance that allows for counseling, sometime soon, it would be an excellent idea to seek some therapy. You have been through a great deal of trauma and no doubt you will be in shock for quite awhile. It is early and this is the beginning of a journey. The point and goal for now is keeping you and yours safe.

7

Post-Escape Recovery

Now, that you are safe, your recovery and healing is most important.

But, I want to acknowledge a few key notes on why leaving the abuser is so difficult and dangerous for the victim of a narcissist. This is something many will never understand unless they have stood in our shoes and lived the life we have lived with a narcissist. The love-bombing, mind-twisting, gaslighting, blackmailing, soul-crushing devaluation, and mental abuse happens like a death by a thousand cuts, not an instant bludgeoning. It comes on slowly and gradually only after the victim cares for and loves the narcissist which ensures that they cannot see clearly. Leaving a narcissist is often seen as not only easier, but truly the only effective way to extricate from this type of abuser. And it is most often recommended to leave rather than expect the narcissist to recover, become enlightened, see the error of their ways, or get over their narcissism and this is due to several key reasons:

1. Lack of Self-Awareness: Narcissists typically lack insight into their behavior and rarely acknowledge their flaws or the impact they have on others. This makes it difficult for them to recognize the need for change.

2. **Resistance to Change:** Narcissistic traits are deeply ingrained and often rooted in early life experiences. Changing such fundamental aspects of personality requires significant effort and willingness, which many narcissists are unwilling or unable to invest.

3. **Manipulative Behavior:** Narcissists often use manipulation, gas lighting, and other tactics to maintain control and protect their self-image. This makes the recovery process complicated and unpredictable, as they may resist or undermine efforts to help them.

4. **Emotional Toll:** Engaging with a narcissist can be emotionally draining and damaging. Their need for admiration and lack of empathy can lead to a toxic dynamic that is harmful to the mental health and well-being of those around them.

5. **Inconsistent Motivation**: Even if a narcissist shows some willingness to change, their motivation can be inconsistent. They might seek therapy or self-improvement for a short period, but without sustained commitment, long-term recovery is unlikely. In fact I would be willing to bet if a narcissist suggested they were willing to seek treatment, there is a high probability it is simply another manipulative ploy. Remember a narcissist always gets their way.

Given these challenges, leaving a narcissist is often considered a more straightforward and healthier option for one's own well-being.

8

Protecting Yourself from Future Narcissists

When examining your future trying to discern how to protect yourself from associating with future narcissists seems like an impossible task. How does one avoid work colleagues, potential future romantic partners and even new friends that all may have narcissistic characteristics in their personality? Most of us are naturally attracted or at least drawn to the narcissist for any number of reasons. We may have been raised by a narcissistic parent and so when we meet a narcissist, even on a subconscious level, we may not realize initially that they are actually a narcissist, but they seem and feel familiar for reasons we may not even realize. Unfortunately, we may also become involved with a narcissist if we act too early and we do not take the time to discern and we just may not see that a person is dangerous for us, until it's too late. Because of this reason alone, we must educate and heal ourselves first. It is also helpful to remember a few important things. The development of narcissistic traits or Narcissistic Personality Disorder (NPD) is influenced by a combination of genetic, environmental, and psychological factors. Understanding what key factors make up the narcissist is critical in understanding what to look for and avoid.

Here are some key factors:

1. **Genetics**: There is evidence suggesting a hereditary component, where individuals may inherit traits that predispose them to narcissism. Again, chances are that a narcissist has more than one factor so I would not get too focused on the genetic factor.

2. **Early Childhood Experiences**: Excessive pampering, overindulgence, or conversely, neglect and abuse during childhood can contribute to the development of narcissistic traits. Inconsistent or excessive praise or harsh criticism can also play a role. Certainly a healthy curiosity about the way someone has been raised can give you a hint about where land on the spectrum of early childhood parenting when they were a child.

3. **Parenting Styles:** Parents who excessively idolize or criticize their children may foster a sense of grandiosity or inadequacy, both of which can lead to narcissism. Again, this comes from learning about one's background, whether they are becoming a new friend, or potential romantic partner.

4. **Cultural and Social Influences:** Societal values that emphasize individual achievement, wealth, and appearance can encourage narcissistic behaviors. It will not take you long to see what another person's priority is when you employ careful observation and listening skills. Use your gut and intuition.

5. **Psychological Factors:** Underlying issues such as low self-esteem, insecurity, or a need to feel special can drive narcissistic behaviors as a the narcissists may over compensate by behaving special, unique, or with a sense of entitlement, even arrogant or haughty, as a front.

***Note these factors often interact in complex ways, making it difficult to pinpoint a single cause for narcissism, therefore it is typically believed that the narcissist seems to possess multiple factors within their make up.**

Most importantly, remember that the narcissist is an expert at holding things together and ingratiating themselves to a potential victim until they have their grips in you. Once they believe you have fallen for them, then their mistreatment will begin. Typically once this starts it is too late or much more difficult to back out of the relationship, even if it is just a friendship, because of the natural dynamics of how the narcissist and the victim/empathic relationship function.

WHO IS IMPACTED BY NARCISSISM AND WHO DOES THE NARCISSIST ATTRACT?

Narcissism primarily impacts those who are in close relationships with the narcissistic individual, such as family members, romantic partners, friends, and coworkers. The specific ways in which these individuals are affected include:

1. **Family Members**: Parents, children, and siblings may experience emotional abuse, manipulation, and a lack of empathy from the narcissistic individual. This can lead to long-term psychological trauma and strained family dynamics.

2. **Romantic Partners**: Partners often endure manipulation, emotional abuse, and a constant need to cater to the narcissist's demands for admiration and validation. This can result in significant emotional

distress and erosion of self-esteem.

3. **Friends:** Friends may feel used, undervalued, or manipulated as narcissistic individuals often seek friendships that provide them with status or admiration.

4. **Coworkers:** In the workplace, narcissistic colleagues or superiors may engage in manipulative or exploitative behaviors to advance their own status, often at the expense of others. This can create a toxic work environment and lead to significant stress and job dissatisfaction.

Overall, the targets of narcissistic behavior are those who are in close, ongoing contact with the narcissistic person, making them vulnerable to the negative effects of such relationships.

Building a Life of Healthy Relationships

In the journey of healing from narcissistic abuse, one of the most crucial steps is to learn to recognize and cultivate healthy relationships. This chapter will guide you through identifying the characteristics of healthy versus unhealthy relationships, setting boundaries, recognizing red flags, building resilience, developing self-awareness and self-care practices, and strengthening your support networks.

Recognizing Healthy vs. Unhealthy Relationships

The first step in fostering healthy relationships is understanding the difference between healthy and unhealthy dynamics. This awareness will help you make informed decisions about who you allow into your life.

Healthy Relationships:

- **Mutual Respect:** Both parties respect each other's boundaries, opinions, and individuality.
- **Trust**: Trust is established and maintained through honesty and reliability.
- **Open Communication:** Both individuals feel safe expressing their thoughts and feelings without fear of judgment or retribution.
- **Equality**: Power and control are balanced. Both individuals contribute equally to the relationship.
- **Support**: Each person supports the other's personal growth and well-being.
- **Empathy**: Understanding and sharing each other's emotions.

Just this is a great checklist... make sure that your relationships have these qualities and you should be pretty solid.

Unhealthy Relationships:

- **Control**: One person seeks to control or manipulate the other.
- **Lack of Trust:** Frequent dishonesty or secrecy that undermines trust.
- **Poor Communication**: Inability to openly discuss issues or feelings.
- **Imbalance of Power:** One person dominates or consistently has more power in the relationship.
- **Neglect or Abuse:** Emotional, physical, or psychological abuse.
- **Lack of Support:** One or both individuals do not support each other's

personal growth or well-being.

If any of these qualities are present in a potential friend or romantic relationship, this is not a healthy relationship and should be avoided at all cost.

Characteristics of Healthy Relationships

Understanding the specific characteristics of healthy relationships can help you build and maintain them in your life. Here are some key traits to look for:

1. **Respect**: Both parties show genuine respect for each other's thoughts, feelings, and needs.
2. **Trust**: There is a foundational trust built on honesty and integrity.
3. **Healthy Communication**: Open, honest, and respectful communication is consistent.
4. **Boundaries**: Each person respects the other's boundaries and personal space.
5. **Mutual Support:** Both individuals actively support and encourage each other's goals and dreams.
6. **Conflict Resolution**: Disagreements are resolved through healthy, constructive discussion without resorting to blame or aggression.
7. **Individuality**: Both individuals maintain their own identities, hobbies, and friendships outside the relationship.

Setting Boundaries and Recognizing Red Flags

Setting and maintaining healthy boundaries is essential for protecting

yourself from potential narcissists and other toxic individuals. Here's how to set effective boundaries and recognize red flags:

Setting Boundaries:

- **Know Your Limits:** Understand what you are comfortable with and what you are not.
- **Communicate Clearly:** Clearly state your boundaries to others in a firm but respectful manner.
- **Be Consistent:** Consistently enforce your boundaries. Do not let guilt or pressure make you compromise them.
- **Self-Respect:** Respect your own needs and limitations. Do not feel obligated to meet others' expectations at the expense of your well-being.

Red Flags:

- **Disrespect for Boundaries**: Repeatedly disregarding your boundaries.
- **Manipulation:** Using guilt, pressure, or deceit to control you.
- **Lack of Accountability:** Refusing to take responsibility for their actions or blaming others.
- **Jealousy and Possessiveness**: Excessive jealousy or possessiveness that limits your independence.
- **Inconsistent Behavior**: Extreme mood swings or unpredictable behavior.

Building Resilience

Building resilience is vital for recovering from narcissistic abuse and protecting yourself in future relationships. Resilience allows you to bounce back from adversity and maintain your emotional health.

1. **Self-Awareness:** Develop an understanding of your emotions, triggers, and responses.
2. **Positive Self-Talk**: Replace negative thoughts with positive affirmations.
3. **Mindfulness Practices:** Engage in mindfulness exercises such as meditation, deep breathing, or yoga to stay grounded.
4. **Healthy Lifestyle:** Maintain a balanced diet, regular exercise, and adequate sleep.
5. **Goal Setting:** Set achievable goals that give you a sense of purpose and direction.
6. **Flexibility**: Learn to adapt to change and accept that not everything will go as planned.

Developing Self-Awareness and Self-Care Practices

Self-awareness and self-care are foundational to maintaining your well-being and building healthy relationships.

Self-Awareness:

- **Journaling**: Write regularly to explore your thoughts and emotions.
- **Therapy**: Seek professional help to understand deeper emotional

issues and patterns.
- **Reflection**: Spend time reflecting on your experiences and what you have learned from them.

Self-Care Practices:

- **Physical Self-Care:** Engage in regular physical activity and maintain a healthy diet.
- **Emotional Self-Care:** Take time to process your emotions and engage in activities that bring you joy.
- **Mental Self-Care:** Stimulate your mind with reading, puzzles, or learning new skills.
- **Social Self-Care:** Maintain healthy social connections and spend time with supportive friends and family.

Strengthening Support Networks

Having a strong support network is crucial for your recovery and ongoing mental health. Here's how to build and maintain these connections:

1. **Identify Supportive Individuals:** Recognize who in your life is truly supportive and positive.
2. **Communicate**: Keep regular communication with your support network. Share your thoughts and feelings openly.
3. **Professional Help:** Seek guidance from therapists or counselors who can provide expert advice and support.
4. **Community Involvement:** Engage in community activities and

build new, healthy social connections.

Embracing Your New Life

Arming yourself with knowledge and tools to recognize healthy relationships, set boundaries, and build resilience, self-awareness, and strong support networks will empower you to protect yourself from future narcissists. Embrace your journey towards healthier relationships with confidence, knowing that you deserve love, respect, and happiness. Your past experiences have made you stronger, and with this strength, you can create a future filled with genuine connections and emotional well-being.

9

Survivor Testimonials

Real-Life Stories of Escaping Narcissistic Relationships

Hearing the stories of others who have successfully escaped narcissistic relationships can provide inspiration, validation, and practical advice. In this chapter, we share testimonials from survivors, real-life stories of escape, the lessons they learned, and their advice for others facing similar situations.

Emily's Story: Rediscovering Self-Worth

Testimonial:

"I was in a relationship with a narcissist for seven years. It started with love bombing, where he showered me with affection and gifts, making me feel like the most important person in the world. But soon, the manipulation and control began. He isolated me from my friends and family, criticized everything I did, and made me feel worthless.

It took me years to recognize the abuse for what it was. The turning point came when I started therapy. My therapist helped me understand that I deserved better and that his behavior was not my fault. With her support, I slowly rebuilt my self-esteem and gathered the courage to leave.

Today, I'm living a life of freedom and self-respect. I've reconnected with my loved ones and am pursuing my passions. My advice to others is to seek professional help and remember that you are worthy of love and respect. Don't let anyone tell you otherwise."

Mark's Story: Reclaiming Independence

Testimonial:

"I was married to a narcissist for twelve years. The relationship was marked by constant gaslighting and emotional abuse. She made me doubt my sanity and isolated me from my support network.

One day, I confided in a close friend who had also experienced a similar relationship. He encouraged me to document everything and seek legal advice. That was the best decision I ever made. With evidence in hand, I was able to secure a protective order and file for divorce.

It wasn't easy, but reclaiming my independence has been incredibly liberating. I now volunteer at a local domestic violence shelter, helping others find their way out of abusive relationships. My lesson is to trust your instincts and reach out for help. There are people and resources ready to support you."

Elizabeth's Story: I Had No Choice but to Escape

Elizabeth had been with Al for a good 10 years and they seemed to have a perfect life, living out in the country. But soon, Elizabeth began to feel more and more isolated losing touch with her friends and family, no longer going out to dinner, traveling, going on dates with her new husband or even making small trips into town anymore. She knew Al liked to drink in the evening, but she didn't see him as a narcissist. Any possible mistreatment she experienced, she always blamed it on Al drinking too much. Still this left her confused and shattered as her self-esteem took one beating after the next as the years went on. As the situation grew more and more intolerable, in a drunken fit, Al pulled a loaded gun on Elizabeth. It was then that she finally realized she was in grave danger and needed to leave. She had no time to make a plan. Elizabeth's advice now is "Always have a plan and don't wait until it is too late or until you are caught off guard. It might be too late to escape. I was blind. I was so use to Al passing out most nights."

Sophia's Escape: Building a New Life

Sophia's relationship with her narcissistic partner lasted for five tumultuous years. The constant emotional manipulation left her feeling trapped and hopeless. One day, a chance encounter with an old friend opened her eyes to the reality of her situation. With her friend's encouragement, Sophia began to plan her escape.

She secretly saved money, sought legal advice, and found a safe place to stay. On the day she left, she felt a mix of fear and relief. The journey was challenging, but with the support of friends, therapy, and legal assistance, Sophia managed to rebuild her life. She now runs a support group for survivors of narcissistic abuse, helping others find their strength and voice.

David's Story: Rebuilding from the Ground Up

David's partner, Lisa, seemed perfect in the beginning. But soon, her true nature emerged, characterized by intense jealousy, control, and emotional abuse. David felt his self-worth eroding daily.

David's Testimonial:
"It was a slow realization that I needed to leave. Lisa's constant belittling made me feel small and insignificant. A friend recommended a therapist who specialized in abusive relationships. Therapy helped me understand the abuse cycle and gave me strategies to rebuild my confidence.

I started setting small goals for myself, like finding a new place to live and reconnecting with friends I had lost touch with. Each step was a battle, but I eventually managed to leave and start anew. Rebuilding my life has been challenging, but every day I feel more like myself."

Lessons Learned and Advice:

- **Therapy is Crucial**: Professional therapy can provide essential tools and strategies for recovery.
- **Set Small Goals:** Breaking down the process into manageable steps can make the overwhelming task of leaving more achievable.
- **Reconnect with Loved Ones**: Rebuilding your support network is vital for emotional strength and recovery.

Lessons Learned and Advice for Others

The journeys of these survivors highlight several key lessons and pieces of advice for anyone seeking to escape a narcissistic relationship:

1. **Seek Support:** Whether through friends, family, support groups, or professionals, having a support system is crucial.
2. **Educate Yourself:** Understanding narcissistic behavior and your legal rights can empower you to take informed actions.
3. **Set Boundaries:** Establishing and maintaining clear boundaries is essential for protecting your well-being.
4. **Plan Your Escape:** If possible, prepare a detailed plan that includes financial, legal, and practical steps.
5. **Rebuild Your Identity**: Engage in activities and relationships that help you reconnect with who you are outside the relationship.
6. **Be Patient with Yourself**: Healing is a gradual process. Celebrate small victories and be kind to yourself along the way.

These personal stories of escape serve as a testament to the strength and resilience of those who have faced and overcome such challenging circumstances. By sharing their experiences, these survivors offer hope and guidance to others on the path to freedom and healing.

10

Legal and Practical Considerations

Legal and Practical Considerations

Escaping a narcissist often involves complex legal and practical challenges. This chapter will touch on helping you understand your rights, the legal protections and resources available to you, how to navigate the legal system, manage shared responsibilities, co-parent with a narcissist, and handle shared assets and finances. It is by no means all-inclusive.

Understanding Your Rights

Knowing your rights is the first step in protecting yourself legally and practically. Each jurisdiction has different laws, so it's essential to familiarize yourself with the specific regulations in your area. This was mention in the first section of the book as well.

1. **Personal Safety:** You have the right to live free from abuse. Laws exist to protect you from physical, emotional, and psychological

abuse.

2. **Legal Representation:** You have the right to seek legal representation. An attorney can help you understand your rights and advocate for you in legal proceedings.
3. **Property Rights:** You have rights regarding shared property and assets. These rights vary depending on whether you are married, in a civil partnership, or cohabitation. Some States recognize common law marriage based on the amount of time a couple has lived together, so be aware of this as well.
4. **Child Custody**: You have the right to seek custody of your children and to protect them from harmful environments.

Legal Protections and Resources Available

There are several legal protections and resources available to help you escape a narcissist and rebuild your life.

Protective Orders: Also known as restraining orders, these legal orders can prevent the abuser from contacting you or coming near you.

Domestic Violence Shelters: These shelters provide temporary housing and resources for individuals escaping abusive relationships.

Legal Aid Services: Many communities offer legal aid services that provide free or low-cost legal assistance to those in need.

Hotlines and Support Services: National and local hotlines can provide immediate support, information, and referrals to resources.

Navigating the Legal System

Navigating the legal system can be daunting, but understanding the process can empower you.

1. **Documentation**: Keep detailed records of all incidents of abuse, including dates, times, and descriptions of events. This documentation can be crucial in legal proceedings.
2. **Legal Counsel:** Hire an attorney experienced in family law and domestic abuse cases. They can guide you through the process and advocate on your behalf.
3. **Court Proceedings**: Be prepared for court appearances and understand what to expect. Your attorney can help you prepare your case and present evidence.
4. **Mediation:** In some cases, mediation can help resolve disputes without going to court. However, this may not be suitable in situations involving abuse.

Managing Shared Responsibilities

When separating from a narcissist, managing shared responsibilities can be challenging.

1. **Dividing Household Responsibilities**: Clearly define and agree on who is responsible for what. Put agreements in writing if possible.
2. **Temporary Arrangements:** Establish temporary arrangements for housing, finances, and childcare until permanent agreements can be made.
3. **Professional Help:** Consider hiring a professional mediator or counselor to help negotiate shared responsibilities amicably.

Co-Parenting with a Narcissist

Co-parenting with a narcissist requires careful planning and clear boundaries to protect your children and yourself.

1. **Parenting Plan:** Create a detailed parenting plan that outlines custody arrangements, visitation schedules, and decision-making responsibilities. Make the plan as specific as possible to minimize conflicts.
2. **Communication**: Use written communication (such as emails or a co-parenting app) to keep a record of interactions. Keep communications focused on the children and avoid emotional topics.
3. **Boundaries**: Set firm boundaries regarding your interactions with the narcissist. Limit contact to what is necessary for co-parenting.
4. **Professional Support**: Engage a family counselor or therapist to help navigate co-parenting challenges and support your children's well-being.
5. **Legal Recourse:** If the narcissist violates the parenting plan or engages in abusive behavior, document these incidents and seek legal recourse.

Handling Shared Assets and Finances

Dividing shared assets and finances can be one of the most contentious aspects of separating from a narcissist.

1. **Financial Documentation**: Gather all financial documents, includ-

ing bank statements, tax returns, and records of shared assets and debts.

2. **Asset Valuation:** Get professional appraisals for significant assets such as real estate, vehicles, and valuable personal property.
3. **Legal Guidance:** Work with an attorney to understand your rights and obligations regarding shared assets and debts. They can help negotiate a fair division.
4. **Financial Independence**: Open separate bank accounts and establish your own credit to gain financial independence.
5. **Debt Management:** Develop a plan to address any shared debts. Be clear about who is responsible for which debts and ensure agreements are documented legally.

Final Thoughts

Understanding your rights, legal protections, and available resources is crucial in escaping a narcissist and protecting yourself from future abuse. By navigating the legal system effectively, managing shared responsibilities, co-parenting thoughtfully, and handling shared assets and finances prudently, you can rebuild your life and ensure a safe, healthy future for yourself and your loved ones. Remember, seeking professional legal and emotional support is essential throughout this process. You are not alone, and help is available.

11

Conclusion

As you reach the end of this journey through understanding and escaping narcissistic relationships, it's crucial to reflect on the importance of self-love and self-respect. These are not mere buzzwords but the foundation of a healthy, fulfilling life. When you love and respect yourself, you set a powerful precedent for how others should treat you. This self-love is your armor against those who seek to diminish your worth. At the same time when you grow up as a child of a narcissist it can sometimes make it difficult to see and recognize anything different. Better the devil you know and see and recognize clearly. But the point is, that we need to recognize that we are worthy of better and we are worthy of love and respect and trust and genuine organic commitment at the soul level without fear of manipulation or being conned or set up or taken advantage of only to be devalued and gaslit and exploited once we let our shoulders down.

Remember, seeking help and support is a sign of strength, not weakness. Whether it's through friends, family, support groups, or professional counselors, surrounding yourself with people who truly care about your well-being is essential. You deserve to be supported, and loved and reaching out for help is a critical step in your healing process.

If you have children, protecting them from the toxic influence of a narcissistic relationship is paramount. They rely on you for guidance and safety. By taking the courageous steps to remove yourself from harmful situations, you also shield them from long-term emotional and psychological damage. Modeling healthy relationships and boundaries will teach them invaluable lessons about self-worth and respect. Attempting to teach them these healthy boundaries early may be the only real way to circumvent the possibility of them falling into the trap of seeking similar relationships in the future or mimicking the behavior of a narcissistic parent.

Finally, begin to speak out about narcissistic abuse. Sharing your story can be a powerful act of liberation and can inspire and educate others. By breaking the silence, you contribute to a broader awareness and understanding of narcissistic abuse, helping to dismantle the stigma and isolation that often surrounds it. It is not just about being selfish or self-absorbed. It is much more than that. It is a manipulative act, that is about power and control. It is also quite cruel and has lasting psychological impact on its' victims. Still if one has never encountered the narcissist personally, they are and remain clueless when trying to understand the survivor of one. Your voice though, can be a beacon of hope and a call to action for those still struggling in the shadows.

In closing, always remember that you are worthy of love, respect, and most of all happiness. Your journey towards healing and self-discovery is ongoing, and every step you take out of the fog is a victory. Embrace the future with hope and confidence, knowing that you have the strength and resilience to build a life free from the shadows of narcissistic abuse. It is not your fault. You will recover. You will always be stronger than you once were. You are brave. I wish you peace and healing.

If you found this book helpful, please consider leaving a review on Amazon.

Thank you.

I was inspired to write this in the aftermath of my own escape from my narcissistic/alcoholic (ex)-husband. And I write it as my own way to break the silence and stigma of being a daughter of a narcissistic Mother and a once-wife requiring an escape plan from her narcissist husband.

There is peace out here.

Be brave.

12

Resources

Pre-Escape Resources

Helpful Contacts and Organizations:

1. National Domestic Violence Hotline (USA): 1-800-799-7233 (SAFE)
2. Women's Aid (UK): 0808 2000 247
3. RAINN (Rape, Abuse & Incest National Network): 1-800-656-4673
4. National Coalition Against Domestic Violence: https://ncadv.org/

Websites and Support Groups:

-Psychology Today: https://www.psychologytoday.com/us/therapists/domestic-abuse

-Loveisrespect: https://www.loveisrespect.org/

-Support Groups for Survivors of Narcissistic Abuse (Facebook, Meetup):

- Facebook Groups: "Narcissistic Abuse Recovery Group"
- Meetup: "Narcissistic Abuse Recovery Support Groups"

Recommended Reading and Further Learning:

1. "The Verbally Abusive Relationship" by Patricia Evans
2. "Why Does He Do That?" by Lundy Bancroft
3. "Psychopath Free" by Jackson MacKenzie

(Please also refer to my entire list of references for some of the very best resources on the topic of narcissistic abuse and recovery)

Post-Escape Resources

Hotlines and Websites:

1. Domestic Violence Hotlines (USA): 1-800-799-7233 (SAFE)
2. Safe Horizon: 1-800-621-HOPE (4673) | https://www.safehorizon.org/
3. National Alliance on Mental Illness (NAMI):1-800-950-NAMI

(6264) | https://www.nami.org/

- Suicide Prevention Lifeline: 1-800-273-8255 | https://suicidepreventionlifeline.org/

Support Groups:

1. Survivors of Incest Anonymous (SIA): https://siawso.org/
2. Narcissist Abuse Support: https://narcissistabusesupport.com/
3. Al-Anon Family Groups (for those affected by another's drinking,

often overlapping with narcissistic behavior): https://al-anon.org/

Recommended Reading and Further Learning:

1. "Healing from Hidden Abuse" by Shannon Thomas
2. "Whole Again" by Jackson MacKenzie
3. "Out of the Fog: Moving From Confusion to Clarity After Narcissistic Abuse"

by Dana Morningstar

Books, Articles, and Research on Narcissism and Recovery:

1. "The Body Keeps the Score" by Bessel van der Kolk
2. "Disarming the Narcissist" by Wendy T. Behary
3. Articles from the Journal of Interpersonal Violence and the Journal of Trauma & Dissociation (Taylor & Francis online)

Resources for Young Children Victimized by Parental Narcissistic Abuse:

1. Childhelp National Child Abuse Hotline: 1-800-422-4453 | https://www.childhelp.org/

2. Children of Narcissistic Parents Support Group (Facebook): "Children of Narcissistic Parents"
3. Books for Children:

- "A Terrible Thing Happened" by Margaret M. Holmes
- "When My Parents Forgot How to Be Friends" by Jennifer Moore-Mallinos

Conclusion

Equipping yourself with the right resources is crucial for both pre and post-escape phases of leaving a narcissistic relationship. Reach out to those that understand, educate yourself, and connect with supportive communities to ensure you and your loved ones are safe, well informed, and empowered with all you need on this journey to safety and recovery. Remember that it is not uncommon for the narcissist to have other addictive behaviors as well, so there are resources that may appear to address issues other than just narcissism for that reason.

13

Appendix

Are You Being Abused by a Narcissist?

Checklist (1+ may indicate narcissistic behavior)

- Do they frequently belittle or demean you?
- Do they lack empathy for your feelings and needs?
- Do they manipulate situations to make you feel guilty or responsible for their actions?
- Do they have an excessive need for admiration and validation?
- Do they lie, cheat, or betray your trust repeatedly?
- Do they isolate you from friends and family?
- Do they react with rage or silent treatment when confronted or challenged?
- Do they project their faults or behaviors onto you?
- Do they make you doubt your perception of reality (gaslighting)?
- Do you feel a persistent sense of fear, anxiety, or helplessness around them?

Evaluating Risks and Safety Concerns

Checklist (even 1 may indicate a serious threat of danger)

- Do they have a history of physical violence?
- Have they threatened you or your loved ones?
- Do they monitor your movements, communications, or finances?
- Are there weapons in the home?
- Do they have access to your personal information, such as passwords or bank accounts?
- Do they have a substance abuse problem?
- Do they display erratic or unpredictable behavior?
- Are there children or pets that could be used to manipulate or control you

Bug-Out-Bag (Items You Will Need)
Checklist

- Personal identification (ID, passport, birth certificate)
- Important documents (medical records, financial documents, legal papers)
- Cash and/or bank cards
- Medications and prescriptions
- Keys (house, car, work)
- Clothes and personal items for you and your children
- Mobile phone and charger
- Sentimental items (photos, jewelry)
- A list of important contacts (friends, family, support services)
- Emergency contact information
- A hidden or secondary phone if possible

How to Create a Safety Plan

Checklist

1. Identify a Safe Place: Know where you can go in an emergency, such as a friend's house, family member's home, or a shelter.
2. Have an Escape Route: Plan the safest way to leave your home. Know which doors, windows, stairwells, or elevators to use.
3. Keep a Bag Packed: Store it in a hidden but accessible place. Include essentials like clothes, documents, money, and medications.
4. Memorize Important Numbers: Have a list of important contacts and keep a copy in your bag.
5. Change Passwords and PINs: Update all your passwords and PINs to something the abuser cannot guess.

6. Secure Your Communications: Use a phone that the abuser does not have access to. Clear browser history and avoid shared devices.
7. Inform Trusted People: Tell friends, family, or neighbors about your situation and ask them to call the police if they hear suspicious noises.
8. Legal Protection: Obtain a restraining order if necessary and keep a copy with you at all times.
9. Children's Safety: Teach your children how to call 911 and identify a safe place they can go in an emergency.
10. Pets: Arrange for pets to stay with a trusted friend or relative if you cannot take them with you immediately.

Self-Assessment Questionnaire

Relationship Health

1. **Emotional Health:**

- Do you feel happy and content most of the time?
- Do you often feel anxious, fearful, or depressed?

2. **Self-Worth:**

- Do you feel valued and respected in your relationship?
- Do you often feel unworthy, undeserving, or inadequate?

3. **Social Connections:**

- Do you maintain healthy relationships with friends and family?
- Do you feel isolated or cut off from your support network?

4. **Boundaries**:

- Are your personal boundaries respected?
- Do you feel your boundaries are frequently violated?

5. **Autonomy**:

- Do you have control over your own decisions and actions?
- Do you feel coerced or manipulated into doing things against your will?

6. **Safety**:

- Do you feel safe and secure in your home environment?
- Do you fear for your safety or the safety of your loved ones?

7. **Communication**:

- Can you openly communicate your thoughts and feelings?
- Do you feel silenced or afraid to express yourself?

8. **Financial Independence:**

- Do you have access to and control over your finances?
- Are you financially dependent on your partner?

Answering these questions can provide insight into the health of your relationship and highlight areas of concern that may need to be addressed. If you find that many of your answers indicate a negative or harmful situation, it may be time to seek help and consider creating a safety plan.

14

References

American Psychiatric Association. (2013). Diagnostic and statistical manual of mental disorders (5th ed.). American Psychiatric Publishing.

Arabi, S. (2016). Becoming the Narcissists Nightmare How to Devalue and Discard the Narcissist While Supplying Yourself. New York, NY: SCW Archer.

Behary, W. (2013). Disarming the Narcissist: Surviving and Thriving with the Self-Absorbed. Oakland, CA: New Harbinger Publications.

Cloud, H., & Townsend, J. S. (2004). Boundaries. Grand Rapids, MI: Zondervan.

Cloud, H., & Townsend, J. S. (2016). Safe people: how to find relationships that are good for you and avoid those that aren't. Grand Rapids, MI: Zondervan.

De Bont, J. (Director). (1996). Twister [Film]. Warner Bros. Pictures.

Durvasula, R. (2019). Don't you know who I am?: How to stay sane in an era of narcissism, entitlement, and incivility. Post Hill Press.

Evans, P. (2010). The verbally abusive relationship: how to recognize it and how to respond. Avon, MA: Adams Media.

Hemfelt, R., Minirth, F. B., & Meier, P. D. (2003). Love is a choice. Nashville, TN: T. Nelson.

McBride, K. (2013). Will I ever be good enough?: healing the daughters of narcissistic mothers. New York: Atria Paperback.

Mellody, P., Miller, A. W., & Miller, K. (2003). Facing codependence: what it is, where it comes from, how it sabotages our lives. New York: HarperSanFrancisco.

Scott, R. (Director). (1991). Thelma & Louise [Film]. Metro-Goldwyn-Mayer Studios.

Thomas, S., & Choi, C. (2016). Healing from hidden abuse: a journey through the stages of recovery from psychological abuse. MAST Publishing House.

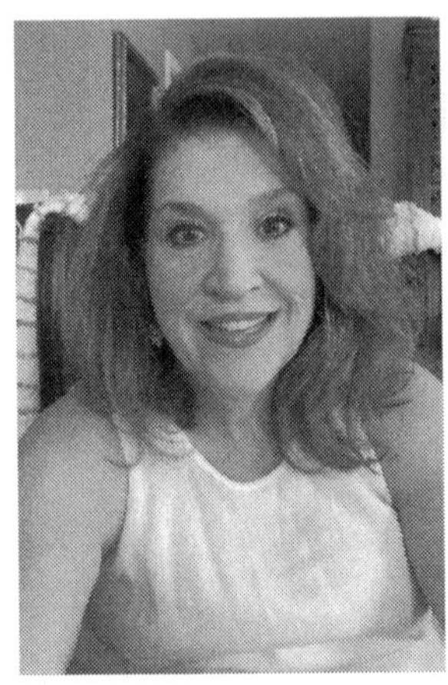

About the Author

Courtenay Beth Bowman is a native Texan who has spent the majority of her career advocating for the rights of women and children. She has a special passion for the voiceless and believes that all individuals have the divine right to be happy, free, and live an abundant life. Her first book, written earlier this year, "Embracing the Divine Feminine: A Guide to Activating Your Inner Power," discusses the transformational process of embracing receptivity, intuition, and authenticity in order to bring balance and harmony back into your life. Ms. Bowman is currently a Women's Empowerment Coach where she helps strong women achieve harmony, confidence and healing peace through self-care and empowerment coaching. She currently resides in a sleepy little town in Southeastern Virginia with her faithful cats, Juno and Bit.

Also by Courtenay Beth Bowman

Learning how to return to the Divinely Feminine in a predominantly Masculine World for balance and harmony.

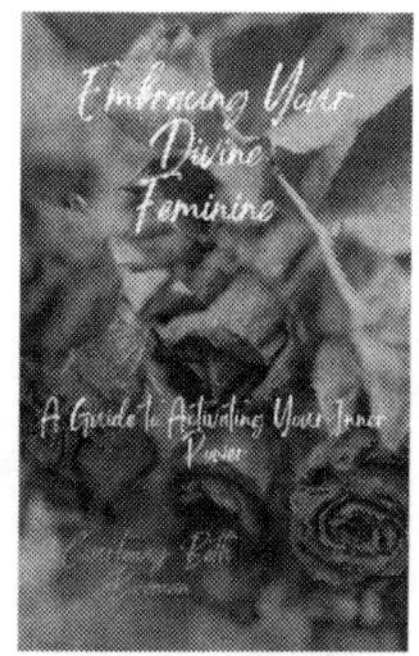

Embracing Your Divine Feminine: A Guide to Activating Your Inner Power

In a predominantly masculine world there is an ongoing journey of resilience and self-discovery. By understanding the challenges, adopting strategies for resilience and embracing authenticity, individuals can navigate societal expectation with grace and strength. The Divine Feminine while a force of transformation, its' essence becomes a guiding light, illuminating a path of empowerment, authenticity, and balance. To truly begin to discover the essence of the Divine, one must launch a valiant exploration of the self, releasing the burdens that inhibit the free flow of authentic expression. And in doing so, shifting from masculine to feminine energy. This is a transformative process that involves embracing receptivity, intuition, and authenticity, but will easily bring balance and harmony to your life.

Made in the USA
Middletown, DE
27 July 2024

57949660R00057